NIGHT
MEDITATIONS

A GUIDED JOURNAL FOR MINDFUL NIGHTS AND RESTFUL SLEEP

ROCK
POINT

Good Evening

As the day begins to fade into the darkness of night, space is created for illumination that comes from within. As we prepare for night, we might find that rather than reflecting on how our inner light shone that day, we run through all of the days concerns, we investigate and analyze, we worry, we pick things apart. Evening teaches us that even as the sky is dark, the stars will shine. There is always light, regardless of what you're going through or how your day transpired. This present moment, this night, is the time to reflect on the good things that happened, let go of the things that no longer serve you, release, and renew.

Underneath the stress and busyness of the day is your calm and natural rhythm. Sometimes it can feel like this rhythm is impossible to access. In the evening, have vast and profound faith in manifesting your desires, surrendering, and letting go. Today is done; tomorrow is yet to arrive.

Consider these moments of quietude before you sleep a time for meditation. Nighttime mediation can calm your anxious mind, soften that inner voice, relieve tension and relax the body, and promote peace. When done before bedtime, meditation can help reduce insomnia and help you look forward to the day to come with confidence and a fresh perspective.

Worry eats up precious time from the things that actually matter and prevents us from focusing on our best selves. Behind the anxiety are beautiful things waiting to be discovered. Find relief from every day troubles by taking time to be in the present moment and close your days with gratitude.

Peaceful Intentions for Restful Nights

This journal contains seasonal meditations to help you unwind and reflect as you wrap up your busy day. Each meditation is followed by writing prompts that will help you dig deeper into your thoughts, feelings, dreams, and personal growth. Each prompt is meant to guide you into nurturing your authentic self through reflection, visualizing your dreams for the future, letting go of what's holding you back, and calming your anxious mind so you can face each coming day with your inner light shining.

These prompts call for self-examination and intention setting, and are organized by the four seasons—spring, summer, fall, and winter. Evenings look and feel different, depending on the time of year, so it's only fitting that the way you greet them is unique as well. When the night is warm and alive with the sounds of summer, you might find that you have a more positive outlook and may use that time to focus on things like gratitude. But when the world outside your bed is frigid and unhospitable, you might take this opportunity to invite in new perspectives.

This journal embraces and encourages all that you are, your brightest inner light. Visiting these meditations each evening is an act of self-love: a way to help yourself gain perspective, give and receive love, and discover more about what makes you so valuable. May your sleep be sound and may peace transcend your worry. Good night.

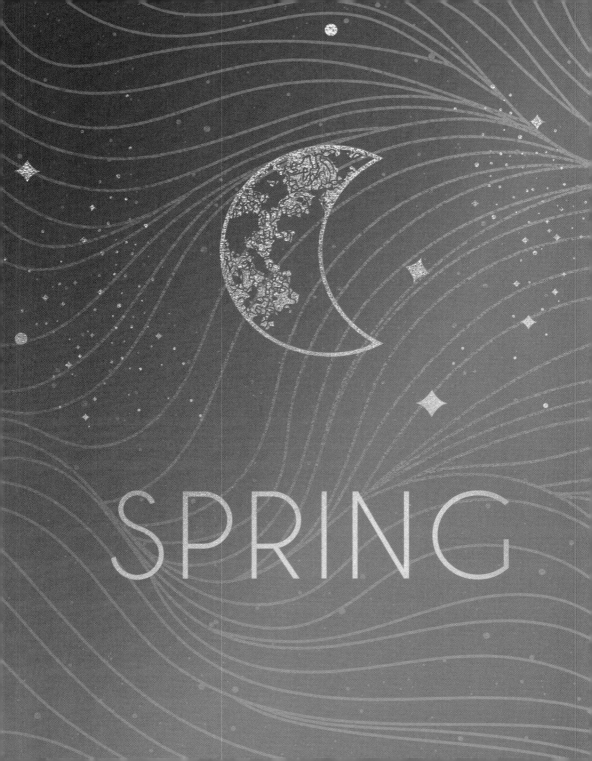

SPRING

Spring is the time when the ground has thawed after the cold of winter. The soil is tilled and ready for the planting of seeds. Creating an environment conducive to growth is necessary for the seeds' success. As spring arrives, think about the seeds you would like to plant in your life and then create an environment for growth. If there is anything you need to let go in order for your seeds to thrive, now is the time to release and plant them. This is the season when we take time to rid our closets and homes of clutter that accumulated during the winter. Spring cleaning creates the sense of a blank slate and starting anew. It is important to do the same for our minds and bodies. We can accumulate clutter spiritually and physically through emotions we have held on to, beliefs that no longer serve us and negative eating habits that need amending. Take note of what is sprouting in your life. Soon the seeds you planted will come to fruition. This is the time to make sure that no weeds are growing where you intended seeds to take root. Let go of what impedes growth. Water your intentions with gratitude and purpose. Be open to receive the rain of blessings that will fall.

There is a plan for your life.
Nothing is a mistake. What comes
next will be revealed in due time. Surrender to
the unknown. It is not necessary to know
everything at all times. Let go of any expectations
and attachments to the outcome. The only thing
that is important right now is this moment.
Be present and breathe peace into the unknown.
Exhale all stress and anxiety. Don't resist
the process; trust the process.

What expectations and attachments do you need to let go of?
If you were to release them, how would your life improve?

....
....
....
....
....
....
....
....
....
....
....
....
....
....
....
....
....
....
....

Fog rolls in and veils the
sun before the last rays of the day.
Through the veil, light can still be seen,
but it appears dimmer. Even though the fog
creates a visual barrier, the sun's rays are still
powerful and light infiltrates the cover. When we go
through ambiguous times, it can feel like we're in
a fog. Although we would prefer to have a clear
picture, the answer is hidden. Allow the light to
shine on the situation. Just as fog
eventually rolls away, so will the
answer be revealed.

Write about a time when you were your true, authentic self.

The manifestation of something we desire is more joyful when it is realized. Setting intentions communicates our deepest desires to the universe. When the moon is full, we can notice what is becoming illuminated in our lives. Look back on the past few months and recognize any desires that have manifested. Acknowledge the work you completed to help this happen and notice how the universe played a part in delivering your intentions. Offer gratitude for both parts working together in the actualization of your dreams.

Write a letter to yourself 5 years ago. Describe how you got to where you are today and who helped you along the way. Close the letter by describing where you'll be in 5 years.

One of the greatest gifts we can give to each other is to listen. Sitting with someone and really taking the energy to listen with love and compassion is an art and a gift. Think of a time when you felt that someone truly listened to you. Remember how it felt to be truly heard. To extend this gift, we need to open our hearts and ears to hear the other person without interruption. Think of one person you can extend this gift to and visualize yourself creating a sacred place for this to happen.

Recall a time when you've been a less than effective listener. In what ways can you improve?

Like a soothing lullaby, the rain falls
onto the roof. As it beats down, it creates a
rhythm. Each drop has its place in nature's
orchestra. The tiniest raindrop makes a difference
to nature's lullaby. If you are feeling small and
insignificant, think about each raindrop. You are
just as important to the rhythm of life. Without
your contribution, the song would be missing
a beat. You are not only a part of the song;
your life is a song.

What are three thoughtful things you can do tomorrow to make someone's day, no matter how small?

....

....

....

....

....

....

....

....

....

....

....

....

....

....

....

....

....

To trust is to let go and know
that everything is working out just
the way it needs to be. This can be a scary
concept, especially when the urge to control
is strong. The key is to release your attachment
to the outcome and have faith that all the work
you have been doing will pay off. Sometimes
the answers are not what we would like to
hear, but they only bring us closer
to where we need to be.

What is one thing you lose sleep over? How would it make you feel to let it go? What are 3 things you can do to help you move toward letting it go?

Our thoughts have a lot of power and positive or negative thoughts affect our attitudes. Think about times when your thoughts were flooded with positivity. Do the same about times when your thoughts were mainly negative. The way to train our minds to stay positive is to catch the negative thoughts when they arise. Stop the thought and reframe it into something positive. Slowly, this process can change the way you think and even react.

What negative thoughts do you repeat to yourself? How can you reframe those thoughts to make them positive?

Spring is the time when the ground has thawed after the cold of winter. The soil is tilled and ready for the planting of seeds. Creating an environment conducive to growth is necessary for the seeds' success. As spring arrives, think about the seeds you would like to plant in your life and then create an environment for growth. If there is anything you need to let go in order for your seeds to thrive, now is the time to release and plant them.

Identify the 'weeds' in your garden. Write about ways that these take up space in your life, and how you can make room for new growth.

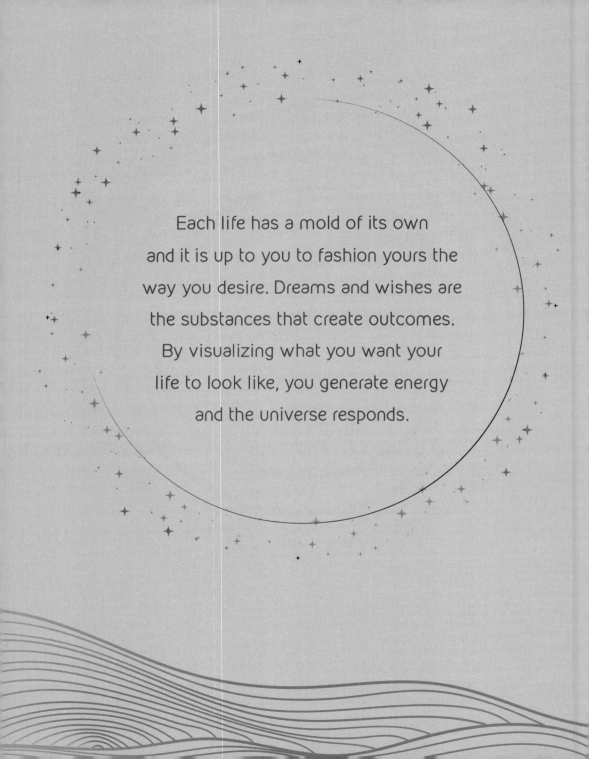

Each life has a mold of its own
and it is up to you to fashion yours the
way you desire. Dreams and wishes are
the substances that create outcomes.
By visualizing what you want your
life to look like, you generate energy
and the universe responds.

Imagine what your perfect day would look like. In detail, describe everything from the moment you wake up in the morning until you close your eyes at the end of the day. Write this in the present tense, as if it were happening now.

The moon wanted to learn to
dance, but being so large, it thought
dancing was impossible. It rotated around the
Earth and watched people dancing in its silver light.
One day the moon looked down over the ocean
and noticed its reflections swaying in the waves. It's
unlikely partner, the ocean, complemented the moon's
desire to dance. The waves moved according to the
moon's pull. Not all partnerships are what we
might have imagined. Keep your heart open
with acceptance and gratitude.

Reflect on a time when an unexpected someone helped you
through a tough situation. What did you learn about yourself?

Dreams can be attained if we believe. Once there were no footprints on the moon or flags on top of Mount Everest. Someone dreamed of these feats and actualized their dreams with hard work and determination. Whatever your dream is, it too can happen. Visualize yourself as if the dream has already come true. Drift off to sleep with this vision in your mind's eye.

If you believed anything was possible, how would your life be different?

Creativity resides in each and every one of us. It takes shape in countless forms and manifests itself in many ways, including through word, song, invention, and artwork. Creators must let go of control to allow their muse to visit and inspire. Creativity thrives in release and contracts with control. To find your creative flow, release your grasp on the outcome. Trust the process and allow inspiration to have its way. Remove restrictions and feel free.

Write about what inspires your creativity. What prevents your creativity from flowing?

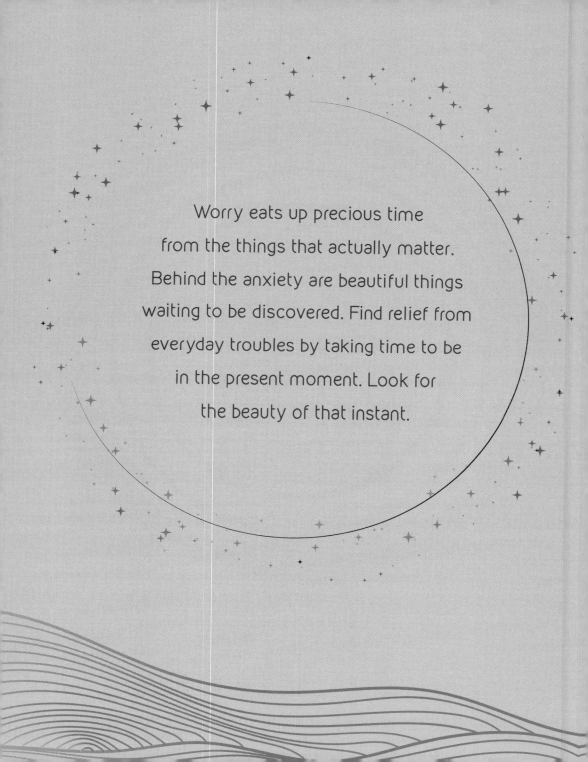

Worry eats up precious time
from the things that actually matter.
Behind the anxiety are beautiful things
waiting to be discovered. Find relief from
everyday troubles by taking time to be
in the present moment. Look for
the beauty of that instant.

Describe 3 positive things that happened or beautiful things that you saw today. Be as detailed as possible.

Noise stimulates and awakens
the senses. Slumber requires silence and
calm. It is important to silence the body
and mind before going to bed. Create the time
to quiet the mind and breathe in and out. Let the
breath calm your body from head to toe.
Scan your body and notice any places
that need extra calming breaths; send
stillness to them.

What are some ways you can re-write your bedtime routine to pave the way for a restful night?

Restless nights can rob us of sleep and fill us with stress. When restlessness occurs, write down what is worrying you to remove the thought from actively working in your mind. After you have recorded these thoughts, let them go. Breathe in calmness instead of worry and drift back to sleep.

Write down the lyrics of a song that makes you feel happy. What good memories does this song trigger?

Our inner lights are
beacons that attract things
to our lives. When we allow outside
influences to affect our ability to shine, we may
believe that our lights are dimmer than they actually
are. But the light still shines. The only thing that can
affect our lights are our thoughts and how we perceive
ourselves. If we allow another person's thoughts
or opinions to contribute to our self-doubt, our
lights dim. Take inventory of your thoughts,
notice where you are doubting yourself,
and shine love into that space.

What is your inner critic saying about you? Write a positive reply to every criticism.

There is so much power in our
heart centers, where love resides. When we
are balanced, we exude generosity, love, and
compassion. When we deny these key functions
of the heart, jealousy, bitterness, and fear take
their place. The universe provides an example of
unconditional love. When we strive to offer this to
ourselves and others, our love and compassion
grow. Visualize a beautiful green light shining
from your heart outward, first surrounding
yourself and then others. Allow the light
to embrace all things.

Who is someone who loves you unconditionally? Describe why you deserve to be loved in this way by them.

Our dreams are powerful and create an energy exchange between our brain and the universe. When we believe in our dreams manifesting, we intentionally set the stage for dreams to actualize. A dream is just the beginning: a spark. From this spark, wonderful things can take place. Believe in your dreams. Embrace them and see where they lead. Nothing is too big if you have trust.

List 10 goals that you would accomplish today if you knew you couldn't fail. What fearless steps would you take to accomplish them?

Feelings of defeat create despair, which can be difficult to let go of. To overcome self-defeat, be your own inner hero. Write down the thoughts that are cultivating defeats, and then rewrite the narrative from a more compassionate point of view. Stop the negative thought loop by creating a positive spin. Reroute the thoughts and tell fear to move aside. When fear and defeat speak, respond with compassion and love.

What healthy daily habit can you start for self-care?

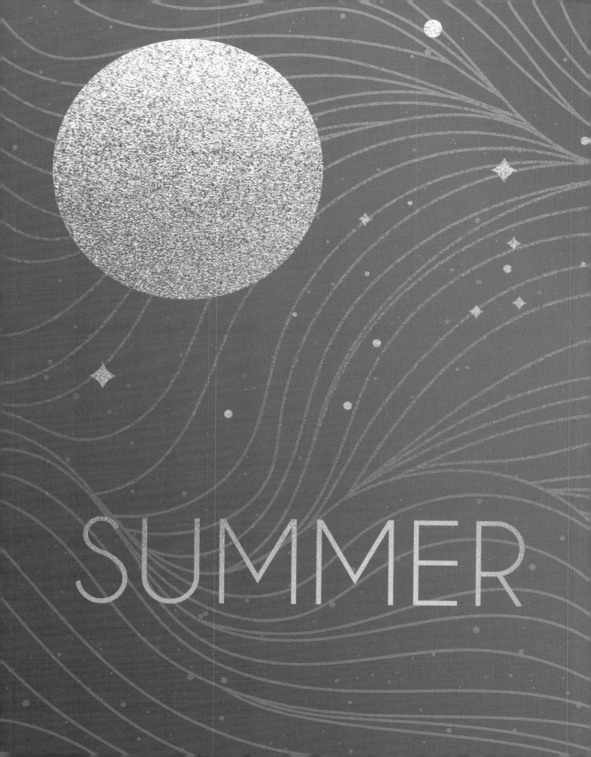

In the driest environment, a yucca shoots up to the sky and blooms brightly. Its yellow and white blooms breathe energy, color, and vibrancy into the desert landscape. Yuccas show that even in a harsh, parched environment, blooming is possible. If you are going through a particularly difficult time, find an opportunity to reach up and thrive. Being mindful of the pain and allowing growth to take place creates resilience. Resilience breeds strength, which moves us forward. A garden that has been neglected has hardened soil, dead plants, and overgrown weeds. A beautiful garden can grow again. Breaking up the dry, cracked ground and removing the dead plants and weeds is just the first step. Our hearts and souls are like gardens. If we neglect them, care needs to occur. Break the hardness up with love and kindness. Find the dead growth and let go. Pull the weeds that hold you back. Growth is on its way.

When we chase things, they
can seem perpetually just out of reach.
There is an illusion of control in the chase.
But the more we try to control, the less
control we actually have. When we let
things go, what we are searching for
has the freedom to appear
or even return to us.

Describe a situation, person, or experience that no longer serves you. If you were to let it go, how would you feel?

Having immediate answers would be wonderful because there would be no room for ambiguity. But if the truth were revealed and all were known, there would be no room for wonder. Allow the spaces of not knowing to create a beautiful anticipation of truth. Even there, magic and wonder can be found. Embrace the unknown with the hope of being dazzled.

How do you currently cope with uncertainty? What are some new, healthy ways you can cope?

Gratitude is the most important prayer of the day. Offering gratitude expresses the acknowledgment of the beautiful things in life. The ability to find things to be grateful for during difficult times strengthens spiritual muscles and attracts more things we can be grateful for in our lives. Take a moment to reflect on the day and express gratitude for the bright spots and opportunities for growth.

Write a list of 10 things or people you take for granted. How can you express gratitude for these?

An artist's hands mold a pot
from a lump of clay. With care, each
turn of the wheel gets the clay closer
to the potter's vision. Afterwards, the artist
puts the pot into a kiln. Through shaping and
fire, a beautiful creation emerges from a lump
of clay. Sometimes we need fire to enhance
our beauty. Remember that in the end,
we can emerge as beautiful vessels
if we are malleable like clay.

Reflect on a difficult situation you've been through. In what ways are you grateful it occurred? What did you learn from it?

What did you think about all day?
Think about any patterns that recur.
Are your thoughts fixated repeatedly on the
same things? If there is something you want
or are striving to become, spend some time
visualizing that. Direct your thoughts toward
the things you want rather than the things
you do not want. Our thoughts
control our focus.

What are 5 ways that negative thinking has an impact on your goals and relationships? Write a positive affirmation that you can use to replace the negative thoughts when they infiltrate your day.

Peace comes from within.
Understanding comes from lessons
learned. During times of unease, know
that a new understanding is forming.
The process is continuous, fluid, and ever
changing. It is important to stay open and
allow each experience to flow as needed.
Search for the meaning in stillness.
There, peace will sprout.

In detail, name 5 things you can see. Name 4 things you can hear.
Name 3 things you can feel. Name 2 things you can smell.
And name 1 thing you can taste.

We may not know what the future holds,
but possibility and wonder are waiting to be
discovered. Don't stop searching for the beauty
in life. Always look for ways to find the incredible
and lovely in every day. You can always discover
something, whether it is external or internal.
When you identify the wonder of the day,
offer genuine gratitude.

Describe your favorite mundane moment of your day today.

Waiting is difficult,
especially when what you are
anticipating feels important. Rest in
knowing that the universe unfolds at just
the right time. When you feel the pang
of longing, breathe into the peace that
everything is being taken care of.
Clarity is on its way.

Describe how impatience makes you feel emotionally and mentally.
What are 3 ways you can help yourself to be more patient?

A still mind is quiet despite the
endless loop of everyday noise. In stillness,
answers are revealed and breath finds the
rhythm of the heart. Letting go of thoughts
and surrendering into stillness creates the space
for revelations and understanding. Getting in
sync with the universe can happen when we
open our minds in quiet and listen
to the voice within.

Choose a single positive word that you want to focus on while you ready yourself for rest, such as love, courage, or gratitude. Write about ways that you have experienced this word and ways that you can make it active in your day tomorrow.

Waiting for answers can
make us anxious and impatient.
In the space of waiting is the opportunity
to be blank and open. Patience allows;
anxiety pushes. Stay open and allow great
things to come your way. Don't force or try
to control them. Everything happens at
just the right time. Rest in knowing
that timing is everything.

Think of a problem that has been causing you anxiety. Describe it as you would to a confidant, then give yourself honest advice.

We can try to plan every detail of our lives, but something can always get in our way. Taking risks requires faith and trusting that you have the resources to overcome obstacles. You can always find ways to gather what you need along the way. But the outcome will never be known unless you take that first step. Leap—and trust that the universe has your needs covered.

What is something in your life that you feel scared to do?
What is stopping you and what are some ways you can overcome
the blockage?

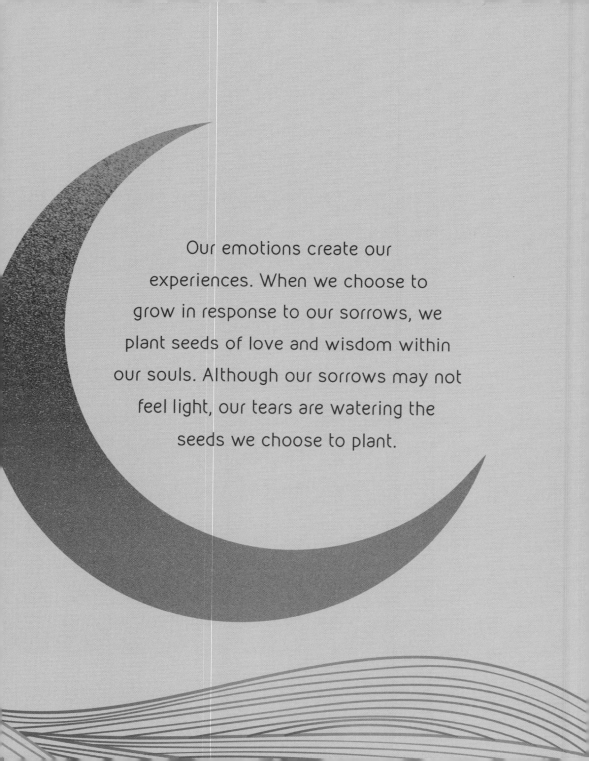

Our emotions create our experiences. When we choose to grow in response to our sorrows, we plant seeds of love and wisdom within our souls. Although our sorrows may not feel light, our tears are watering the seeds we choose to plant.

Who or what most helps you get through difficult times?

Living in the past allows yearning to
take hold of our hearts. We may reference
supposed glory days as a standard, but then
we forget that in fact the greatest things lie ahead
of us. Focus on the present moment instead of
ruminating on the past or projecting into the future.
What we create right here, right now, molds
what is next. Seize this moment while
having gratitude for the past.

Reflect on a teacher or a mentor who made a positive impact on your life. Write about specific ways they improved your life or outlook.

Sleep is not instantaneous.
We cannot expect to be busy and
preoccupied right before we go to sleep.
We must ease ourselves into calm and peace,
so as not to muddy it with half-finished tasks
and half-thought ideas. Tonight, ease into bed
one step at a time. Take a moment to meditate
and clear your mind of nagging cares.
Then, get ready for sleep.

Describe 5 ways that you can adjust your nightly routine in order to lay the groundwork for a truly restful night.

Letting go of the past is a difficult process, but if we held on to each thing we have ever been attached to, the weight would be too much to bear. There is freedom and lightness in releasing what no longer fits into our lives. When old patterns, relationships, and clutter are cleared out, we make space for growth and for new things to enter our lives. Make room for what is to come by releasing your grasp on the past.

What expectations of others can you let go of?

Waves ripple gently along
the shore of the bay. The sky turns
from soft pastels to deeper, darker hues
of the night. Peace and quiet abound. The
day is done; all is well. Our thoughts are like
the waves, slowly rippling in and out. When
we desire peace, we can replace negative
thoughts with a simple mantra to
coincide with our breath: "I am calm.
I am at peace. I am at rest."

Write your own serenity mantra in such a way that you will use it in
your daily life. Repeat your mantra to yourself as you fall asleep.

Invite peace to enter your soul. The day has ended and all of its troubles are over. Take a moment to practice this breathing exercise before you fall asleep: Breathe in peace; breathe out worry. Breathe in peace; breathe out dangling thoughts. Breathe in peace; breathe out stress. Breathe in peace and allow all tension to slowly leave your body, from your head to your toes.

In what ways are you currently experiencing anxiety in your body? What can you physically do before bed to help relieve this tension?

In the midst of stillness, vibrancy is restored. Finding quiet in chaos allows you to recharge your inner glow. Learning to be still is a practice that reaps great rewards. Just like a good night's sleep delivers vitality for the day ahead, stillness restores mind, body, and soul. Embrace stillness to shine a little brighter.

Where is your "happy place"? Describe it in detail, along with all of the feelings it brings to you.

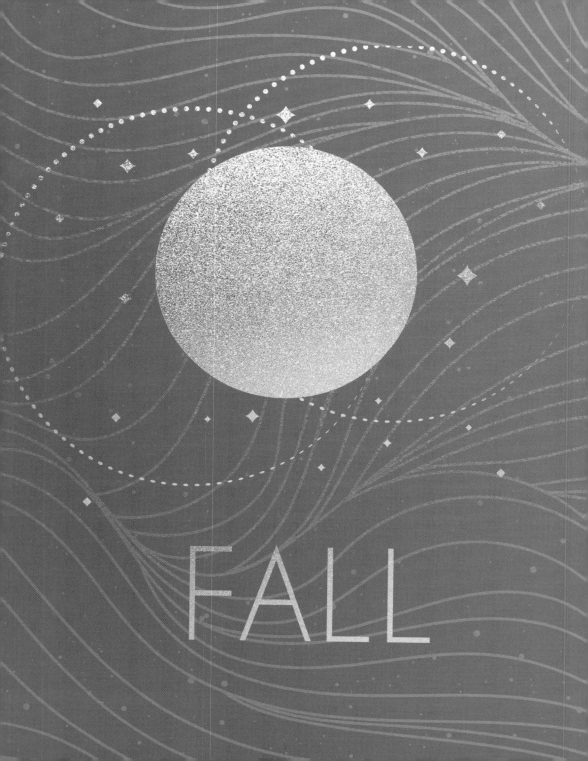

As the season turns from summer to fall, the leaves change colors on trees, adding brightness to a cooler environment. Before they fall, golden leaves—the final burst of sunny color—are a reminder of the summer's vibrancy. When the final leaf falls, the tree becomes dormant in preparation for the winter. This is the perfect time to reflect on your vibrancy. Even during transitions, we emit light. When the evening air becomes crisp in autumn, the harvest is almost complete. Fruit and grain are gathered after a bountiful growing season. The work of pruning in the spring and tending in the summer determines the quality of the crop. At times, there are plants that will not produce, so they are no longer tended to. If there is something that does not promise growth, focus elsewhere. Reaping what we sow also applies to the attention that we give.

Heaviness weighs down the soul. Negative emotions bring the soul's vibration down and positive emotions lift them. When there is heaviness in our hearts, a positive thought can alleviate the weight of the intense emotions. Before you drift off to sleep, do a smiling meditation. Close your eyes and smile, taking deep breaths through the nose. Revel in the lightness.

Write about 5 small things that bring you joy.

When the day is complete,
we turn off the lights as we prepare
for bed. The space becomes dark and our
senses adjust. When darkness takes over, we
cannot rely on our sight. We must use our other
senses a bit more to compensate. At times we
feel off and find ourselves overcompensating
as a reaction. But if we allow the natural
adjustment to take place, we can find our
balance more quickly.

Describe a situation in which you felt completely balanced and calm.

Deep in the sea, a school of fish gathers and swims with fluid ease. As the fish ride the currents, they find a natural and communal rhythm. In a group they find security traversing the ocean. Our community can be a place of safety and camaraderie. Think about your community this evening and offer gratitude for every member. Notice where the movements of your group are fluid and where you may need to make adjustments. Visualize fluid movements as if you are all riding an ocean current.

When was a time that your community was a support system
for you?

During the strongest winds, the branches of a tree sway, giving in to the wind's influence. Down on the ground, the trunk stands firm with its roots reaching into the earth, allowing the branches the freedom to sway. Like a tree, we can find stillness through the changes in life. It is important to stay grounded and find our inner stillness to help get through such times. Find your center and allow stillness to calm and ground you.

What makes you feel safe, supported, and at peace? What are some
ways you can include this in your daily life when you feel most
stressed or overwhelmed?

Bright in the sky, the
moon shines down, providing light
for the harvest. Hard work and patience
are rewarded as farmers reap what they sowed
in the spring. It is time to reflect on how your
seeds have developed. Harvest is the culmination
of growth and pruning. Appreciate the work
that this harvest provided. Be grateful for your
patience and perseverance. Breathe in this
contentment and allow your dreams to
revel in this harvest.

Write about a time when you accomplished something by laying solid groundwork and allowing it to grow. Reflect on how your patience paid off.

Expectations lay a foundation
for disappointment. We can
accomplish great things when we
measure without expectations. Let go
of the outcome and see the positive
in all things, no matter how great
or small. Wonderful things are
happening all around us.

What impossible standards are you holding yourself and others to? What are some ways you can begin to release those expectations?

Sit quietly and exhale all
the stress from the day. Seek the
messages that wait in the stillness.
We are connected to the stars and the
wind. Locate the place where your intuition
resides. Ask a question that is on your mind
and wait for the answer. Let go of your
timetable. The answer will appear
when the timing is right.

If you can't change your current situation, what is one thing you can do to move in the right direction?

We always have a chance to begin again. Let go of whatever happened today, knowing that tomorrow is new and full of opportunity. Allow yourself to become still and to breathe in this moment. Notice any tension you may be holding on to and breathe soothing breaths into that space. Let the breath melt the tension from your body and feel yourself becoming lighter in the stillness.

Describe a mistake that you learned from. How has that lesson improved your life?

Silence is healing and can be more powerful than noise. In outer space, there is a void where stars, planets, and moons revolve around the sun. The solar system demonstrates the ability to orchestrate without sound. The most powerful forces in nature coordinate to make this silent symphony take place. If the solar system can operate in silence, we can take a lesson and harness the power of silence. Create a space of sacred silence and just be.

What ways can you change your daily routine to allow for moments of silence? Write a challenge for yourself, like limiting social media time or other distractions.

Time slips by
without notice when we spend
our days in a rush. Taking moments
to practice mindful awareness creates a
sense of pause and calm. Breathe into beautiful
moments to take in the sights, sounds, smells,
tastes, and feelings they bring. Make mental
notes of where you experience awe. Pause in
awe. These moments are gratitude generators.
Contemplate the beautiful moments of the day
and appreciate the awe they provided. Then,
breathe in the current moment and
recognize its beauty.

What are 3 beautiful things you saw or heard today? What are 2 pleasant things you smelled today? What is 1 thing you enjoyed tasting today? How did you feel in these moments?

Kindness creates
connection and healing. Our
words and actions are products of
our hearts and soul. What we think and
feel manifests outwardly. If you experienced a
moment of kindness today, breathe in the fullness
of that joy. Remember how it felt to give or
receive that kindness. Deposit the feeling into your
memory bank so that you can recall it later. Kind
thoughts produce kindness. The more we
contemplate good things, the more we
will exude goodness.

Recall an act of kindness that you've received. What are some small ways you can pay it forward this week?

During a storm, a snail emerges, moving slowly to avoid drowning. It is not worried about the rain or its pace; it just continues to move forward. Even at the risk of exposure to predators, snails move without fear. When life feels stormy, keep moving forward. One small step each day can create the momentum you need while the storm passes. Don't allow fear to paralyze movement. Keep going, because storms always pass.

When something negative happens, what are some traits or skills that you already have that can help you face fear and find the positive?

A lotus radiated beauty and noticed how people stopped to admire it. The lotus worried that the admirers would be alarmed if they knew that every night, it descended into the mud only to return the next day. Perfectionism can create discontentment and judgment. What others don't see does not affect them. Self-judgment removes joy from situations where love and acceptance await. Accept what is and offer love and gratitude to those places where acceptance is needed. Without the mud, the lotus would not be as radiant.

Who are your role models and heroes? In what ways are you
like them?

To love someone means
that you do not expect anything
in return. Love is one of the most basic
human needs. We desire the love of others
and when our hearts are open we wish to give
love. Keeping the heart open is essential to nurture
and extend love. What's most important is to
give this gift to ourselves. When we can love
ourselves, we can love others. As you fall
asleep, reflect on all of the things you
love about yourself.

Write a love letter to your body, thanking it for all that it does for you every day.

A hardened heart
can soften again with enough
care and love. Trials and fire soften
some of the hardest and densest materials
and souls. Forgive and heal whatever caused the
hardness. Allow grace to enter the space that
has atrophied. Let grace permeate the space
and slowly reveal and soften the core where
love and understanding reside. In this space,
forgiveness and love can return and
heal. Embrace the release.
Soften into restoration.

Think of something that you need to forgive yourself for. Write down the reasons why you need to release this and how forgiving yourself will promote healing.

Things come to an end for a reason. Death is not only an ending but also a beginning. When a flower dies, it falls to the ground and creates room for another bloom to occur. If something in your life is ending, let go and make room for what wants to come. Open your heart and mind to whatever is next. The pain of the ending will pass and the beauty and joy of a new beginning will replace it.

Describe a time when you cleaned out a closet space, the garage, your car, or your home. Think of things that were difficult to throw away. How did you feel once the job was done and the space clean?

....

....

....

....

....

....

....

....

....

....

....

....

....

....

....

....

....

Every snowflake is different
and significant. Each one eventually
delivers water to streams and lakes. We
can behold wonder and beauty in such a small
thing. Each human is different and significant
as well. Each person has a purpose and a soul.
Looking for the beauty in every person we meet
fosters acceptance and tolerance. Offer the
love and appreciation you desire to others.
Genuinely embrace differences. Where
there is acceptance there is peace
and understanding.

What is something about someone in your life that is difficult for you to accept? Write about ways that accepting them would make a positive impact on your life. How will it make a positive impact on theirs?

The art of doing nothing
cultivates great understanding. When
our minds are full of thoughts and our days
are busy, understanding does not have room
to expand. Find some time each day to stop for
a few minutes to breathe and clear space. When
you first wake up, take five breaths to ground
yourself. In the middle of the day, take five
breaths to regroup. At the end of the day,
take five breaths to calm down. Extend
the stillness as time goes on.

What are some small shifts you can make in your day to create space for moments of reset?

Imagine that you
are near the beach and the
water is calm and warm. Walk out
into the ocean and notice how clear the
water is. There is soft white sand at your
feet and warm turquoise water all around. Lie
back into the sea and face the sun. Allow the
saltwater to hold your body. Float effortlessly.
Feel the gentle sway of the water creating
immense calm within. As you close your
eyes in bed tonight, recall this image
and fall into a deep sleep.

Write about a memory of a time you felt perfectly safe, warm, and content. Go into as much detail as possible, describing all five senses.

WINTER

To prepare for the bareness of winter, a beaver gathers and builds a safe, warm place. Many animals collect their reserves for hibernation. This is the time for preparation and planning. What are you preparing and planning for? If you would like to get something done, create a plan. Allow your dreams to take place in this sacred space. Don't force anything. Breathe in this openness and breathe out worry. Everything will fall into place. This season reminds us that the vastness of space is a place where anything is possible and galaxies exist. Comets fly, planets orbit the sun, and stars are born. Creating spaciousness in our minds and in our physical environments makes room for stillness and peace. We can realize and actualize greatness in the space of stillness. A quiet mind is like a clean, blank page. Contemplate possibility. Allow dreams to take place. There are no boundaries where creation awaits.

A moth's activities are
conducted at night. The moth navigates
using the moon's light. Naturally attracted to
light, moths are drawn to lamps and fires as well.
Their attraction to light makes them seem mysterious
when they appear from the dark. They bring with
them vital nectar to pollinate plants and flowers to
help keep nature's balance. The light guides them
and helps their journey. Even when the moon
is new, a moth always finds light to
help it on its way.

If you could spend a day doing only things that made you feel happy and relaxed, what would those things be? How can you work 2 of those things into your day tomorrow, even in the smallest way?

Night has fallen, the stars
appear, and the moon creates a silver
glow. It is time to rest and renew the mind.
Find inner calm by shutting down all devices
and giving the body and mind the time to slow
down and ease into a restful state. Release
everything that happened today. Let go of
tomorrow's plans. Set the stage for dreams
to occur. Anything is possible
in this calm state.

Time for a Worry Dump: Without pausing too long to think, write down everything that comes to mind that is worrying you. Do this for 5-10 minutes, then release them to the page.

I release all the stress from the day and allow calm
to permeate my soul. As I breathe in, I bring peace
and tranquility to the places that feel tense. As I exhale,
I let go of the tension, stress, and frustration. I welcome
quiet and surrender any noises in my mind. Rest is the
state I am about to enter. Dreams and restoration will
come to me in sleep. I breathe in restoration
and breathe out the rest of the day.

Think about your personal mantra and use this to set your intention for tomorrow.

In the darkness of night, a nightingale
sings its song. He waits for the perfect time
to sing—without the noise of other birds—and
sings a song for dreamers. Its melody stirs
creative potential within the dreamer and
releases the mind from the day's troubles.
The song is a lullaby that accompanies the
shining of the stars. The moon creates a
spotlight for the night's song and
accompanies it with peace.

What is your creative outlet? What are some ways you can make time to engage it more frequently?

The beauty of the present moment
is that the past is a teacher and the future is
a dream. The ability to be right here, right now
is a practice. When the lessons or dreams seek
attention in the present moment, acknowledge their
presence, but let them flow away for they do not
have a place right now. Release attachment to
outcomes of the past and future and breathe into
this moment. Notice something lovely in your
surroundings. Pay attention to your breath.
Be grateful for the quiet moment you
have created for yourself.

Describe 5 things you are grateful for and why.

Coral is the skeletal outside of tiny sea creatures; it also creates a home for fish and provides protection for them to hide from predators. The reefs produce a colorful underwater shelf displaying a rainbow of colors. But coral is sharp, and if touched, inflicts pain. The dichotomy of providing protection while inflicting pain highlights its dual nature. Duality exists in all things and we have the power to choose how we perceive them. Perception shapes our reality. Choose to focus on beauty.

Reflect on a situation that was unexpectedly difficult for you.
List 5 "silver linings" that came from it.

Slumber descends. The body relaxes deeply, releasing all of the tension from the day. There is nothing that needs to be done, no words left to speak. The moon is high in the sky and the stars are dancing in her iridescent light. Lights are dim and the darkness envelops its surroundings like a peaceful hug. Calmness and tranquility manifest through our breath. Dreams unveil themselves from thoughts that are now asleep. Rest takes over.

What does being perfectly relaxed look like to you?

A lighthouse provides a
guiding light for ships at sea. Its light
shines in darkness, through fog, and during
storms. Your inner light is your beacon through
the dark times in life. To access your light, close
your eyes, sit quietly, and listen to your breathing.
Allow all thoughts to fade away. In stillness,
your light can illuminate the truths that noise
sometimes overwhelms. Like a ship coming
safely to harbor, your soul will find
peace in the darkness.

Describe a moment in nature when you saw something seemingly glowing from within? How did it make you feel?

Have vast, profound faith
in manifesting your desires. Allow
your dreams to take place; trust the
universe with them. As you fall asleep, set
an intention, release it to the universe, and
be patient. Forces beyond your control are
taking care of you and working to help
you manifest your desires. Surrender
and let go. Breathe in peace;
breathe out control.

Using careful detail, describe what your perfect life would look like today. Write it as if it is currently happening.

Hush now. As quiet envelops
the night, it's time for slumber and
dreams. In silence, our inner wisdom finds
its voice. Connect with this silence and let go
of your thoughts. You don't need them right now.
In the void, dreams can take place. In the silence,
ideas take shape. Quiet your mind by breathing
in the silence and breathing out the noise.
Listen to your breath as it goes in and out.
Allow the breath to cover you
in peace and quiet.

Look around you. Describe your surroundings and what you like the most about your space.

The craters on the moon are places of damage, where asteroids hit the moon's surface. These supposed scars create depth and complexity, making the moon even more beautiful. No matter how many scars the moon has, it still reflects the sun's light, illuminating others. Our damage also creates depth and complexity in our souls. The key is to transform the pain into something beautiful. Don't hold on to the scar; let it heal and then appreciate the complexity it provides.

Think about a time that someone hurt you. Write down 2 ways that forgiving them could improve your life and outlook.

Lights begin to illuminate
the city as the sun sets. Only the
brightest stars can be seen among the
sparkle of the city. But all the stars are still
shining. It is easy to allow our light to dim
when we sense the brightness of others. But we
have the power to shine as bright as possible
so that our lights can be seen. Imagine how
illuminated the planet would be if we all
shone as bright as we could.

What are 5 of your most unique talents? How can you apply them, even in small ways, in your daily life?

Worry and fear imprison
the mind. We can become slaves
to the false truths they provide. When
we act out of fear, we are not being true
to ourselves. Write down your fears and
notice where your anxiety is creating
an inaccurate picture of reality.
Identify the truth and embrace
it with peace.

Think of a recent argument you had with a close friend or family member. Describe the situation from the other person's perspective.

Moonlight casts
shadows between the rows of
trees in an orchard. Late at night it is
quiet and peaceful here. The chirps of crickets
interrupt the silence and the stars shine bright
above. The shadows follow the moon as night
progresses. There is nothing to do except be still.
The stillness creates renewal for another day in
the sun and for bearing fruit. But for now,
in this moment, quiet is all that matters.
Tonight, rest is all that matters.

What brings you true joy that money can't buy?

A feeling of discontent can cast a shadow in the soul. Longing for something that we don't have fixes our minds elsewhere. In this state, the shadows can permeate and settle. To counteract this mind-set, practice gratitude. On the hardest days, it is important to find things to be grateful for. Before falling asleep, think of three things you are grateful for today. Continue to think about these things. Allow your final thought of the night to be gratitude.

You've won an award. Write an acceptance speech thanking all of the people who have helped you achieve success.

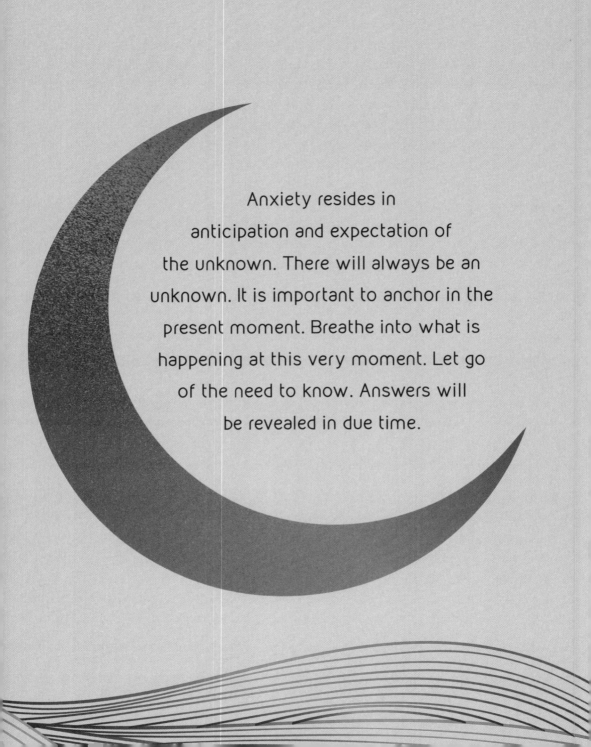

Anxiety resides in
anticipation and expectation of
the unknown. There will always be an
unknown. It is important to anchor in the
present moment. Breathe into what is
happening at this very moment. Let go
of the need to know. Answers will
be revealed in due time.

What would be most helpful to hear when you're feeling anxious and overwhelmed? Write a list of 5 affirmations that are meaningful to you.

The more outer
space is explored, the more
apparent it becomes that we have much
to learn. The universe is vast and our reality is
a tiny dot. This knowledge highlights the grandeur
and greatness of something much bigger and more
powerful than we are. Think about this force and about
any issues that may be flooding your mind. See that
whatever you are going through is an exchange of
energy. Infuse any nervous energy with calm,
healing energy, knowing that the universe
has everything under control.

When did you most recently ask someone for forgiveness?
How has your relationship with them grown since then?

Surrendering to our life's
purpose brings happiness and
contentment. Be open to what life
wants from you. Look for where your soul
lights up and ignites purpose within. Every
person has something they are good at.
Embrace your natural strengths and
the greatness that results.

What ignites your passion?

Brimming with creative inspiration, how-to projects, and useful information to enrich your everyday life, quarto.com is a favorite destination for those pursuing their interests and passions.

This edition published in 2022 by Rock Point, an imprint of The Quarto Group,
142 West 36th Street, 4th Floor, New York, NY 10018, USA
T (212) 779-4972 F (212) 779-6058 www.Quarto.com

Contains content previously published in 2017 as *Moonlight Gratitude* by Rock Point, an imprint of
The Quarto Group, 142 West 36th Street, 4th Floor, New York, NY 10018, USA.

Rock Point titles are also available at discount for retail, wholesale, promotional, and bulk purchase. For details, contact the Special Sales Manager by email at specialsales@quarto.com or by mail at The Quarto Group, Attn: Special Sales Manager, 100 Cummings Center Suite 265D, Beverly, MA 01915 USA.

10 9 8 7 6 5 4 3 2

ISBN: 978-1-63106-876-8

Publisher: Rage Kindelsperger
Creative Director: Laura Drew
Managing Editor: Cara Donaldson
Editor: Sara Bonacum
Cover and Interior Design: Kim Winscher

Printed in China

This journal provides general information on forming positive habits and creating feelings of peace and calm. It should not be relied upon as recommending or promoting any specific diagnosis or method of treatment for a particular condition, and it is not intended as a substitute for medical advice or for direct diagnosis and treatment of a medical condition by a qualified physician. Readers who have questions about a particular condition, possible treatments for that condition, or possible reactions from the condition or its treatment should consult a physician or other qualified healthcare professional.